HUMAN ANATOMY and PHYSIOLOGY
PRACTICAL NOTEBOOK

for

First Year Diploma in Pharmacy

(According to the new syllabus prescribed by the Pharmacy Council of India, Education Regulation 1991, implemented in the year 1993, for Diploma in Pharmacy Students)

Varun Dutt Sharma M. Pharm.
Principal

S.K. Pandey B. Pharm.
Sr. Lecturer

Janta Polytechnic, Jahangirabad, Bulandshahar, Uttar Pradesh

CBS

CBS Publishers & Distributors Pvt. Ltd.

New Delhi • Bengaluru • Chennai • Kochi • Kolkata • Mumbai
Hyderabad • Nagpur • Patna • Pune • Vijayawada

Human Anatomy and Physiology
PRACTICAL NOTEBOOK

ISBN: 81-239-1427-X

First Edition: 2007
Reprint: 2011, 2014, 2016, 2017, 2018, 2019, 2020

Published by **Satish Kumar Jain** and produced by **Varun Jain** for
CBS Publishers & Distributors Pvt. Ltd.,
4819/XI Prahlad Street, 24 Ansari Road, Daryaganj, New Delhi - 110002
delhi@cbspd.com, cbspubs@airtelmail.in • www.cbspd.com
Ph.: 23289259, 23266861, 23266867 • Fax: 011-23243014

Corporate Office: 204 FIE, Industrial Area, Patparganj, Delhi - 110 092
Ph: 49344934 • Fax: 011-49344935
E-mail: publishing@cbspd.com • publicity@cbspd.com

Branches:
- ***Bengaluru:*** 2975, 17th Cross, K.R. Road, Bansankari 2nd Stage, Bengaluru - 70 • Ph: +91-80-26771678/79 • Fax: +91-80-26771680 E-mail: cbsbng@gmail.com, bangalore@cbspd.com
- ***Chennai:*** No. 7, Subbaraya Street, Shenoy Nagar, Chennai - 600030 Ph: +91-44-26681266, 26680620 • Fax: +91-44-42032115 E-mail: chennai@cbspd.com
- ***Kochi:*** Ashana House, 39/1904, A.M. Thomas Road, Valanjambalam, Ernakulum, Kochi • Ph: +91-484-4059061-65 Fax: +91-484-4059065 • E-mail: cochin@cbspd.com
- ***Kolkata:*** 6-B, Ground Floor, Rameshwar Shaw Road, Kolkata - 700014 Ph: +91-33-22891126/7/8 • E-mail: kolkata@cbspd.com
- ***Mumbai:*** 83-C, Dr. E. Moses Road, Worli, Mumbai - 400018 Ph: +91-9833017933, 022-24902340/41 • E-mail: mumbai@cbspd.com

Representatives:
- Hyderabad: 0-9885175004
- Patna: 0-9334159340
- Jharkhand: 0-9811541605
- Nagpur: 0-9021734563
- Pune: 0-9623451994
- Uttarakhand: 0-9716462459

Printed at:
J.S. Offset Printers, Delhi (India)

Certificate

Student's Name ______________________________

Class ______________________ Roll No. ______________

This is to certify that experiments, written in the index, have been performed by the student, are satisfactory.

Grade.................. Name and signature of lab. in-charge

College stamp Date ....

Preface

The ultimate objective of technical education is to develop relevant skill, creativity and competancy among the students so as to enable them to perform the task effectively and efficiently later in the world of work. To obtain the above aim, and to reduce the writing work load of the students, this practical notebook of "Human Anatomy and Physiology" for diploma in pharmacy first year has been written according to new syllabus as prescribed by Pharmacy Council of India, education regulation 1991. This practical notebook contains 20 experiments. Left hand side page of every experiment has been left blank for making diagram, calculation and observation.

We shall be gratefully acknowledged the comments, suggestions and criticism by respected teachers and students for improvement of future edition. We express sincere thanks to Mr Satish Kumar Jain and Mr Y.N. Arjuna, M/S CBS Publishers & Distributors for their cooperation, encouragement and assistance in bringing out the present form of this manual. Finally ours greatest gratitude are to our colleagues, friends and family members.

Varun Dutt Sharma • S.K. Pandey

Syllabus

(50 hours)

1. Study of human skeleton.
2. Study with the help of charts and models of the following system and organs:
   (a) Digestive system
   (b) Respiratory system
   (c) Cardiovascular system
   (d) Urinary system
   (e) Reproductive system
   (f) Nervous system
   (g) Eye
   (h) Ear
3. Microscopic examination of epithelial tissue, cardiac muscle, smooth muscle, skeletal muscle, connective tissue and nervous tissues.
4. Examination of blood films for TLC, DLC and malarial parasite.
5. Determination of clothing time of blood, erythrocyte sedimentation rate and haemoglobin value.
6. Recording of body temperature, pulse rate, heart rate, blood pressure and ECG.

Contents

INDEX

S. No.	Name of the experiment	Page No.	Remarks

1 HUMAN SKELETAL SYSTEM: Osteology

Experiment 1

OBJECT

To study the different types of bones of **axial skeleton** of the human.

The axial skeleton can be classified as follow

1. Skull — Cranium and facial bones
2. Vertebral column
3. Sternum
4. Ribs

SKULL

Cranium

(i) It is a large hollow rounded part of the skull. It is formed of 8 flattened bones, i.e. 1 frontal, 2 parietals, 1 occipital, 2 temporals, 1 sphenoid and 1 ethmoid.
(ii) Sutures provide immovable joint which include coronal, sagittal and lambdoid.
(iii) *Frontal bone* forms the roof of the orbit and nasal cavity. It contains supra orbital margin, nasal notch supercilliary arch and frontal sinus.
(iv) *Parietal bones* form the side wall and the roof of the cranium. They are articulated anteriorly with frontal bone, posteriorly with occipital bone and below with the temporal bone.
(v) *Temporal bones* are situated at lateral sides of the skull. The zygomatic process is articulated with zygomatic bone
(vi) *Occipital bone:* It forms the back and lower part of cranium cavity having an opening known as foramen magnum through which spinal cord passes. It is wing-shaped bone at middle part of cranium +containing sella turcica which provides facet for the pituitary gland.
(vii) *Ethmoid bone:* It is cube like bone of it situated between the orbits.
(viii) *Caranium* protects the brain.

Facial bones: These are bones of face and are composed of 14 bones.

Maxillae (Upper jaw) 2	They form the upper jaw. The upper set of teeth are arranged in it. It has a pyramid shaped body and possesses zygomatic, alveolar, frontal and palantine processes.
Mandible (Lower jaw) 1	It is only movable bone of the skull. The lower set of teeth are fixed in it. It contains coronoid process and condyle which is articulated with temporal bone. Facial bones form jaws to support the mouth.
Palatines 2	They form mainly hard palate.
Zygomatic 2	These are cheek bones.
Lacrimal 2	They contain lacrimal sac which secretes the lacrimal fluid.
Nasal 2	They are situated between the socket of eyes.
Inferior nasal chonchae 2	They are found in nasal cavity.
Vomer 1	This vertical bone forms nasal septum.

STERNUM (Breast bone)

1. It is long, narrow, flat and vertical bone in the middle of the front wall of the chest. It has main three parts.
   (i) *Manubrium:* Triangular part bearing clavicular notches on both sides of articulation with clavicle and articular surfaces on both side for the first ribs.
   (ii) *Body:* It provides space for attachment of 3rd, 4th, 5th, 6th and 7th ribs.
   (iii) *Xiphoid bone:* It is lower part of the sternum
2. **Function:** It plays a role in the respiratory mechanism. It also helps in formation of thoracic cage.

RIBS

1. The ribs are curved, movable bones and 12 pairs in number. They are classified depending on their attachment.
   (i) *True ribs:* The upper 7 pairs of ribs are attach directly to the sternum.
   (ii) *False ribs:* The next 3 pairs of ribs are joined to the sternum in directly through costal cartilages.
   (iii) *Floating ribs:* These are the lowest 2 pairs which are free in front.
2. Structure: The rib consists of 2 parts
   (i) *Vertebral part:* It is long and bony which articulates with the thoracic vertebrae by 2 facets, the capitulum and tuberculum (1st nine ribs) and by single facet the head (in the remaining vertebrae)
   (ii) *Sternal Part:* It is short and cartilaginous which articulates with the sternum.
3. Functions
   (i) They protect the heart, lung and kidney.
   (ii) They provide space for attachment of external and internal intercostal muscles.
   (iii) They play an important role in mechanism of respiration.

VERTEBRAL COLUMN

There are 33 vertebrae which are grouped into 5 categories.

Sl. No.	*Type*	*Region*	*No.*
1.	Cervical	Neck	07
2.	Thoracic	Chest	12
3.	Lumber	Abdomen	05
4.	Sacral	Hip	05
5.	Coccygeal (caudal)	Coccyx	04

Atlas

1. It is first cervical vertebra
2. It is also called 'yes bone' as head can nod on atlas forward or backward
3. It lacks a body and spinous process.
4. Neural foramen is divided into upper spinal foramen and lower odontoid canal.
5. Odontoid process is absent.
6. The upper surface has two facets which articulate with the condyles of occipital bone.

Axis

1. It is the second cervical vertebra of vertebral column.
2. It is also called 'no bone' as it supports sideways turning movement of head .

3. Neural spine is present which is small and bifurcated.
4. Neural foramen is not divided
5. Centrum (body) is present which is directed upward.
6. Odontoid process (upward projection of body) articulates with atlas.
7. A foramen on either side is found for the vertebral artery to pass through to the brain, is called foramina transversaria.

Thoracic

1. There are 12 in number.
2. Centrum (body) has facets one on each side for the attachment of head of ribs.
3. Transverse process has also facets for tubercle of rib attachment.
4. Neural spine is long and down ward directed.
5. Vertebral foramen is absent.
6. Transverse process are club shaped.

Lumbar

1. There are five in number.
2. Neural spine is short, flat and upward directed.
3. Facets for rib are absent.
4. Transverse processes are thin and elongated.
5. Body (centrum) is big and kidney shaped.

Sacral

1. There are five in number and all are united to form a single bone sacrum.
2. Sacral foraminae 4 in number through which nerves pass.
3. The sacrum lies between the innominate bones of the pelvic girdle.

Coccygeal Vertebrae

1. These are four in number.
2. They are very small, rudimentary and fused to form a curved triangular bone, the coccyx .
3. The coccyx have no function.

Experiment 2

OBJECT

To study the different bones of **appendicular skeleton** of the human.

APPENDICULAR SKELETON

1. **Girdles**
   (i) Pectoral (Shoulder girdle)
      (a) Scapula
      (b) Clavicle
   (ii) Pelvic (Hip girdle)
      (a) Ilium
      (b) Ischium
      (c) Pubis
2. **Limbs**
   (i) Fore limbs
      (a) Humerus (Upper arm)
      (b) Radius ulna (Fore arm)
      (c) Carpals (Wrist bones)
      (d) Metacarpals
      (e) Phalanges
   (ii) Hind Limbs
      (a) Femur (Thigh bone)
      (b) Tibia fibula
      (c) Tarsals (Ankle)
      (d) Metatarsals
      (e) Phalanges

Scapula

1. *Location:* Posteriolateral region of the thorax.
2. It is a large, flat and triangular bone
3. *Glenoid cavity:* For articulation of the head of the humerus.
4. There are two surfaces, i.e. anterior and posterior which provide fossae for attachment of muscles.
5. There are three angles and three borders
6. *Functions:* It provides articulation to the arm bones. It also provides attachment to muscles of the arm.

Clavicle

1. It is also known as collar bone.
2. It is long and curve bone of shoulder girdle.
3. The sternal end articulates with sternum where as acromial end articulates with acromion process of scapula.

Pelvic girdle

It consists of innominate bones (two) including sacrum and coccyx.

INNOMINATE BONE (HIP BONE)

1. It is made up of three bones, i.e. ilium, ischium and pubis.
2. *Acetabulum:* A deep cup shaped hollow structure where the head of femur fits into it.
3. *Ilium:* The surfaces of ilium provides attachment to muscles (gluteal and iliac). It also contains notch for articulating with sacrum.
4. *Pubis:* It is the front part which contains symphysis pubis (union of the pubic bones), superior and inferior ramus.
5. *Ischium:* It is the lower part containing the body, tuberosity, spine and obturator foramen.
6. *Functions:* It supports and protects viscera. It transfers the weight of body to the leg. It provides attachment to muscles of leg.

Humerus

1. It is a bone of upper arm.
2. The spherical upper part is head which is articulated with glenoid cavity of scapula.
3. The middle long part is called shaft which possesses deltoid ridge.
4. The lower end containing trochlea articulated with ulna having two epicondyles
5. Capitulum articulates with radius.

Ulna

1. It is inner bone of fore arm.
2. Olecranon process and coronoid process are fitted into olecranon fossa and coronoid fossa of the humerus respectively.
3. The shaft of ulna gives attachment to the muscles of fore arm.
4. The lower part of ulna conatins head and styloid process.

Radius

1. It is outer most bone of fore arm.
2. The upper part of radius contains a head, neck and biceps tubercle.
3. The shaft gives attachment to muscles.
4. The lower end of the radius forms wrist joint with three carpal bones.
5. It also forms radio-ulnar joint.

BONES OF WRIST and HAND

Wrist: 8 carpals which are arranged in two rows containing four bones in each row.
1st Row: Scapoid, lunate, triquetral and pisiform.
2nd Row: Hamate, capitate, trapezoid and trapezium.
Palm: 5 metacarpals.
Fingers: 14 phalanges (2 + 3 + 3 + 3 + 3).

Leg bone

Each leg contains 30 bones.

Bone	*Region*	*Number*
Femur	Thigh	1
Patella	Knee	1
Tibia and Fibula	Lower leg	2
Tarsals	Ankle	7
Metatarsals	Sole	5
Phalanges	Toes	14

Femur

1. It is thigh bone which is the longest bone of the body.
2. The head is round and articulates with the acetabulum of innominate bone.
3. The head has body ridges called trochanters.
4. The shaft has no deltoid ridge but contains gluteal ridge and linea aspera.
5. The lower end has two condyles.

Patella

1. It is a sesamoid bone.
2. The posterior surface is smooth.
3. The anterior surface is covered with bursa.
4. It forms knee joint with femur.

Tibia

1. It is the inner most bone of the leg.
2. The upper end possesses a head which articulates with condyles of femur.
3. The shaft is triangular in shape.
4. The lower end takes part in formation of ankle joint.

Fibula

1. It is the outer most bone of the leg.
2. The upper end contains head and styloid process.
3. The shaft gives attachment to muscles.
4. The lower end contains lateral malleolus and malleolar fossa.

2 HUMAN SYSTEMS: Anatomy and Physiology

Experiment 3

OBJECT

To study the anatomy and physiology of **digestive system** with the help of chart and model.

The digestive system comprises the following organs.

1.	**Mouth**	It is mainly made up of vestibule and oral cavity. The oral cavity contains hard palate and soft palate. At middle uvula is located. The important organ of mouth are (i) *Tongue:* It bears taste buds and three types of papillae, i.e. circumvallate, fungiform and filiform. (ii) *Teeth:* The permanent teeth are 32 in number, arranged into rows. Each half of the jaw has 2 incisors, 1 canine, 2 premolars and 3 molars. Each tooth has three parts a crown, a neck and a root. The tooth is made up of a hard material dentine, pulp and the covering enamel. The teeth along with tongue and saliva helps in mastication of food. (iii) *Salivary glands:* There are three pairs, i.e. parotid, submaxillary and sublingual.
2.	**Pharynx**	It is situated between mouth and oesophagus. It consists of nasopharynx, oropharynx and laryngo pharynx . The bolus is passed from oral cavity to oesophagus through oropharynx and air passes from nasopharynx to larynx through laryngopharynx.
3.	**Oesophagus**	A muscular tube-like structure which open in to the stomach. It is situated between trachea and vertebral column. The process of swallowing the bolus takes place here and finally the bolus is carried to stomach.
4.	**Stomach**	It is situated in the upper part of abdominal cavity below the diaphragm. Stomach has two ends, i.e. cardiac and pyloric end; two borders, i.e. lesser curvature and greater curvature and two surfaces, i.e. anterior and posterior surfaces. The cardiac end is guarded by cardiac sphincter where as pyloric end is guarded by pyloric sphincter. The upper part is called the fundus and lower main part is called the body. The stomach secretes gastric juice which contains pepsin, rennin, HCl and intrinsic factor. The condition of the food after digestion in the stomach is called chyme.
5.	**Small Intestine**	It is divided into three parts: (i) *Duodenum:* It is C-shaped tube which receives the bile and pancreatic juice through openings of bile duct and pancreatic duct respectively. (ii) *Jejunum:* It is called middle portion of small intestine. It bears numerous glands which secrete succus entericus juice. (iii) *Ileum:* It is the distal part of the small intestine. Many lymphoid structures are found which are called Payer's patches which provide protection against infection.
6.	**Large Intestine**	(i) *Caecum:* A sac-like structure, right to iliac fossa, is guarded by ileo caecal valve. (ii) *Appendix:* It is blind vestigial organ at ileocaecal valve. (iii) *Ascending colon:* It is situated vertically upward and continue to transverse colon.

(*Contd.*)

(iv) *Transverse colon:* It runs transversely and near the spleen continues to form descending colon.

(v) *Descending colon:* It lies vertically down ward at left lumber region.

(vi) *Sigmoid colon:* It is found in pelvis region and terminates in to rectum.

(vii) *Rectum:* It is found in lower part of pelves and continues into anus. Rectum and anus play an important role in process of defecation.

Physiology of digestion

The process of digestion begins from mouth. Saliva contains ptyalin which acts on starch to form maltose. Maltase again changes maltose into glucose to some extent. Gastrin acts upon gastric glands to stimulate the secretion of gastric juice. The enzyme pepsinogen its converted in to active pepsin by the action of HCl. This pepsin acts on protein to form peptones and proteoses. Rennin converts caseinogen into casein. Casein is digested further by pepsin. The pH of the stomach is acidic. In duodenum bile acts on chyme to make the pH alkaline (pH 7.10 to 8.2) and also emulsifies the fats. The pancreatic juice contains number of enzymes, i e. trypsinogen, chymotrypsinogen, amylase and lipase.

$$\text{Trypsinogen} \xrightarrow{\text{Enterokinase}} \text{Trypsin + Protein = Proteoses + Peptones}$$

$$\text{Chymo-Trypsinogen} \xrightarrow{\text{Trypsin}} \text{Chymotrypsin}$$

$$\text{Protein +} \xrightarrow{\text{Chymo-Trypsin}} \text{Peptides}$$

$$\text{Peptides} \xrightarrow{\text{Peptidase}} \text{Dipeptides + Amino acid}$$

Pancreatic lipase acts on fats to form fatty acid and glycerol. Amylase acts on carbohydrate to form disaccharides.

Hormonal control: Duodenal epithelium secretes 6 hormones.

1. *Enterogestrone:* It inhibits the secretion of gastric juice.
2. *Cholecystokinin:* Causes secretion of bile from gall bladder.
3. *Pancreozymin:* Causes release of enzyme in pancreatic juice.
4. *Secretin:* Causes release of $NaHCO_3$ and pancreatic juice.
5. *Enterocrinin:* Causes release of enzyme from the crypts of Lieberkuhn into intestinal juice.
6. Villikin: Activates the movement of villi.

Intestinal juice from small intestine contains amylase, maltase, sucrase, lactase, peptidase, lipase, nucleotidase which act on starch, maltose, sucrose, lactose, peptides, emulsified fats and nucleotides respectively to form maltose, glucose, glactose, amino acids, fatty acids, glycerol and nucleosides.

Experiment 4

OBJECT

To study the anatomy and physiology of **human heart** with the help of chart and model.

ANATOMY (human heart)

Location	The heart is hollow muscular organ which is located in middle of the thoracic cavity slightly on the left side of the chest.
Protective covering	It is made up of three layers. (i) *Endocardium:* Inner membrane (ii) *Myocardium:* Middle layer. (iii) *Pericardium:* It is outer most layer and is filled with pericardium fluid to protect the heart from mechanical injury and prevent friction.
Chambers	The human heart has four chambers. The right side chambers are right atrium and right ventricle. Similarly left side chambers are left atrium and left ventricle.
Septum	Two atria are separated by inter auricular septum. Where as ventricles (right and left) are separated by inter ventricular septum.
Valves and Apertúres	(i) *Atrioventricular opening:* Opening between right atrium and right ventricle is guarded by tricuspid valve. (ii) *Left atrioventricular apertures:* Opening between left atrium and left ventricle which is guarded by bicuspid valve or mitral valve. (iii) *Semi-lunar valves:* The pulmonary arch and systemic aorta have semi-lunar valves.
Chordae tendinae and papillary muscle	The inner surface of the ventricle has muscular ridges and conical muscular elevations with white tough cords are termed as papillary muscle and chordae tendinae respectively which prevent over distension of the valves (tricuspid and bicuspid)
Blood vessels	(i) *Superior venacava and inferior venacava:* These venacava carry venous deoxygenated blood to the right atrium of the heart. (ii) *Pulmonary artery:* It carries deoxygenated blood to lungs for purification. (iii) *Pulmonary veins:* They carry oxygenated blood to the left atrium of the heart. (iv) *Systemic aorta:* The left ventricle gives of systemic aorta which carries oxygenated blood to the various organs except the lungs.

Function of the Heart

The heart pumps the blood to all parts of the body. The cardiac muscle plays an important role in this process. The heart gets nourishment from coronary arteries which arise from the aorta. The three events take place in a cardiac cycle, i.e. auricular systole, ventricular systole and joint diastole.

The left atrium receives oxygenated blood from pulmonary vein where as deoxygenated blood is supplied to right atrium by superior and inferior venacava. The right ventricle receives deoxygenated blood from right atrium and in the same time the oxygenated blood reaches into the left ventricle from the left atrium by contraction of atria. Now the contraction of both ventricles take place. The deoxygenated blood from right ventricle goes to lungs through pulmonary trunk. The oxygenated blood is circulated to all parts of the body except lungs through systemic circulation.

Experiment 4

Experiment 5

OBJECT

To study the anatomy and physiology of **respiratory system** with the help of chart and model.

Nostrils and nasal cavity	There are two chambers separated by nasal septum. Each chamber opens externally by nostrils. Each chamber has three regions, i.e. lower vestibule, middle respiratory and upper olfactory. The hairs present in the chambers prevent the entry of dust particles. The wall of each chamber has three body ridges called nasal **conchae**. The nasal chambers open into nasopharynx by internal nares.
Pharynx	It has three parts: (i) *Nasopharynx:* It is the upper part. The internal nares open into it. (ii) *Oropharynx:* It is the middle part. (iii) *Laryngopharynx:* It the lowest part.
Larynx	It is more prominent in men than in women. It is short tubular structure and is guarded by cartilages like thyroid, cricoid and arytenoid. It opens into laryngo pharynx by glottis. The glottis bears a cartilaginous flap, the **epiglottis**. During swallowing the epiglottis closes the glottis to check the entry of the food into it.
Trachea, bronchi and bronchioles	Trachea is also called windpipe. It is divided into two tubes called bronchi. One bronchus enters in the right lung and the other in the left lung. The right bronchus is divided into upper, middle and lower bronchi while left bronchus is divided into upper and lower bronchi. The secondary bronchi are subdivided into smaller tertiary bronchi which divide into still smaller bronchioles. The wall of trachea and bronchi bear 16–20 C-shaped incomplete cartilaginous rings to support the walls of the trachea and the bronchi to prevent their collapsing.
Lungs	A pair of lungs are located in the thoracic cavity, laterally enclosed by the ribs and in front by the sternum. They are elastic, spongy and cone shaped organ. The right lung is bigger and is divided into three lobes while left lung is divided into two lobes. Each lobe is made up of lobules which contains bronchial tubes. The bronchi and bronchioles finally end into air sacs or alveoli.
Pleura	Lung is covered by serious membrane call pleura. Pleura has two layers, i.e. the inner visceral layer and the outer parietal layer. The pleural fluid is filled in the space between these two layers.
Diaphragm	It is dome shaped sheath of muscle which separates the thoracic cavity from the abdominal cavity.
Intercostal muscles	These are two types of muscles, i.e. external intercostal muscle and internal intercostal muscle. Both the muscles are arranged between the ribs in the opposite to each other.

Physiology of respiration

Inspiration

It is an active process. The contraction of diaphragm results in lowering of the diaphragm. It means the diaphragm becomes flat. It enlarges the thoracic cavity vertically. The contraction of intercostal muscles pull the ribs and

sternum upward and outward. They enlarge the chest cavity sidewise. The abdominal muscles relax. The lung expands and the pressure in the lung is less than atmospheric pressure so air follows the following route.

External nares → Nasal chamber → Internal nares → Pharynx → Glottis → Larynx → Trachea → Bronchi → Bronchioles → Airsac

Expiration

It is a passive process. It involves relaxation of diaphragm and external intercostal muscles. The diaphragm becomes dome-shaped again. The ribs and sternum return to original position. As a result the thoracic cavity become smaller. The air follows the following route.

Airsac → Bronchioles → Bronchi → Trachea → Larynx → Glottis → Pharynx → Internal nares → Nasal chamber → External nares

Mechanism

Respiration is regulated by nervous and chemical control.

Nervous control

The medulla oblongata contains inspiratory centre and expiratory centre. Diaphragm is innervated through phrenic nerve while intercostal muscles are innervated through intercostal nerve. Inspiratory centre control the process of the inspiration through this nerve while expiratory centre brings about the relaxation of the respiratory muscle and hence controls the process of expiration. Apneustic and pneumotaxic centres are located in the pons of the brain. Stimulation of apneustic centre stimulates respiratory centres. Pneumotaxic centre has inhibitory influence on the apneustic centre.

Chemical control

The chemical regulation is influenced by CO_2 tension of the blood. The increase concentration of CO_2 stimulates the respiratory centre directly. The lack of oxygen for prolong time may result in cyanosis and even death.

Experiment 6

OBJECT

To study the anatomy and physiology of **urinary system** with the help of chart and model.

The urinary system consists of the following organs:

1.	**Kidneys**	There are two bean shaped situated on the posterior wall of upper abdomen. The outer part of the kidney is called cortex. The inner part is called medulla which contains pyramids and calyces. Calyces unite to form pelvis of the kidney. The nephrons are the structural and functional unit of the kidney. A nephron has two part. (i) *Malphigian bodies:* It is made up of Bowman's capsule and glomerulus. (ii) *Renal tubules:* They consist of proximal convoluted tubule, loop of Henle, distal convoluted tubule and collecting tubules. Each kidney has about 1,200,000 nephrons.
2.	**Ureters**	The pelvis of the kidney continues into a tubular structure known as ureter. Both the ureters open in the urinary bladder. The urine formed from the kidney is carried out by ureter to the urinary bladder. The lining layer of the ureter is made up of fibrous and muscular tissue.
3.	**Urinary bladder**	It has muscular sac-like structure. It has two parts, i.e. fundus which is upper part and base which is lower part. It acts as reservoir for the urine. Micturition is mainly controlled by the sphincter and muscular coat of the urinary bladder.
4.	**Urethra**	It is canal like structure continue from bladder to outside. Male urethra is long while female urethra is short.

Physiology

Kidney regulates the water, ion and pH balance. It helps in excretion of waste products and poisonous substances. It also plays an important role in urine formation. The formation of urine involves the following process.

1.	**Glomerular filtration**	This takes place in Bowman's capsule containing a bunch of capillaries called glomerulus. The glomerular filtration rate in normal adult human is about 120 ml per minute. Glomerular filtration rate depends on permeability of the capillaries, area of filtration, osmotic pressure of the blood plasma (30 mm), hydrostatic (20 mm) and intra capillary pressure (75 mm). The net filtration pressure is 75–(30+20). This is called ultra filtration.
2.	**Tubular reabsorbtion**	The glomerular filtration which is about 172 litres daily, passes into tubule. Kidneys excrete only 0.5 to 1.5 litres of urine daily. So the rest amount of filtrate is reabsorbed by the tubules. (i) *Proximal convoluted tubule:* Glucose amino acid, hormones, vitamins, Na^+, K^+, Mg^{++} and Ca^{++} are reabsorbed by active transport. Chloride ions are reabsorbed by passive transport while water passes into peri-tubular capillaries by osmosis. (ii) *Henle's loop:* The first wide part of the descending limb is impermeable ions, urea and water but the narrow part of descending limb is freely permeable to water. Ascending limb of Henle's loop is permeable to inorganic ions. (iii) *Distal convoluted tubule:* Reabsorbtion of water takes place under the influence of ADH by osmosis while Na+ is reabsorbed under the influence of the aldosterone by active transport.
3.	**Tubular secretion**	It occurs mainly by active transport in the proximal and distal convoluted tubules. The materials secreted include creatinine, hippuric acid, K^+, H^+, NH_3 and foreign substances.

Experiment 7

OBJECT

To study the male and female **reproductive system** of human with the help of chart and model.

MALE REPRODUCTIVE SYSTEM

Testes	Two oval testes are suspended in the scrotum through spermatic cords. Each testis is made up of numerous seminiferous tubules which form spermatozoa by the process of spermatogenesis. Interstitial cells (Leydig cells) are found between seminiferous tubules which secrete the hormone testosterone. The cells of Sertoli are present which provide nutrition to spermatozoa. ***Function*** (i) To form spermatozoa (ii) To secrete testosterone (anabolic and sexual role)
Epididymis	The seminiferous tubules form rete-testes which give rise to vasa efferentia. Vasa efferentia join at the upper end of the testes to form epididymis. Seminiferous tubules ⟶ Rete-testes ↓ vasa efferentia ⟶ Epididymis
Vas deferens (2 in numbers)	Epididymis continues into tube like structure called vas deferens. It travels, upwards across abdominal cavity, pelvis part and finally joins with the seminal vesicle.
Seminal vesicle (2 in numbers)	These are secretory glands. Vas deferens join with seminal vesicle to form ejaculatory duct. So ejaculatory ducts are two in number which pierce the prostate gland.
Prostate gland	It is single secretory gland which provides nutritive secretion for spermatozoa. It also secretes prostaglandin.
Penis	It is composed of erectile tissue like corpora cavernosa and corpora spongiosum. The triangular tip of the penis is called glans penis.

Female reproductive system

It consists of the following organs:

External genital organs	These organs are collectively called vulva which include labia majora (outer layer hair covered fold of skin), labia minora (inner small moist thin fold of skin), clitoris (erectile body), hymen and vestibule.
Internal genital organs	1. **Vagina:** It is large muscular tube which open externally by vaginal orifice. The space toward the cervix is called fornix. ***Functions*** (i) It helps in copulation. (ii) It helps in menstrual flow. (iii) It acts as birth canal during parturition.

(Contd.)

Experiment 7

2. **Uterus (womb):** It is elastic pear shaped and muscular organ which is located between the bladder and the rectum. It has four regions.
   (i) The upper dome shaped is fundus.
   (ii) The upper corners are cornua.
   (iii) The middle main part is body or corpus.
   (iv) The narrow lower part is cervix.
   It is made up of three layers
   Outer: perismetrium,
   Middle: myometrium
   Inner: endometrium

   Functions
   (i) It receives the fertilized ovum and forms placenta for the development of the foetus.
   (ii) It helps in menstruation.
   (iii) It helps in expulsion of the foetus.

3. **Fallopian tube (oviducts):** These are muscular tube two in numbers. They have four regions.

   (a) *Infundibulum:* It is broad funnel shaped part which ends in finger like processes called fimbriae. Fimbriae open in to ostium.

   (b) *Ampulla:* The long and wide part.

   (c) *Isthmus:* It is very short, narrow and straight part.

   (d) *Uterine part:* It communicates with the uterine cavity.

   Function: Fertilization of ovum.

4. **Ovaries:** There are two in number and primary female sex organ. They are located in the lower part of abdomen and attach to the broad ligament by the mesovaria. They are composed of connected tissue, the stroma and the outer covering is called germinal epithelium. The stroma consists of two parts:
   (a) *Outer:* Ovarian cortex
   (b) *Central:* Ovarian medulla. The ovarian medulla contains the follicles at various stages of development. The mature Graafian follicle contains an ovum surrounded by many layers of follicle cells which secretes oestrogen in to the blood. When ovum is released from Graafian follicle it forms corpus luteum which secretes the hormone progesterone. If pregnancy does not occur, corpus luteum degenerates to form corpus albicans.

   Functions
   (i) Secretion of oestrogen and progesterone.
   (ii) Formation, maturation and release of ovum.

Experiment 8

OBJECT

To study the anatomy and physiology of **CNS** with the help of chart and model.

The nervous system is of mainly two types:

A. Central nervous system.

B. Peripheral nervous system

The CNS consists of brain and spinal cord. The peripheral nervous system includes cranial nerves (12 pairs) and spinal nerves (31 pairs).

Brain (encephalon)

It is divided in to three regions.

1. **Fore brain (prosencephalon)**

   (a) **Cerebrum:** It is the largest part of the brain. Cerebrum has two equal hemispheres and are joined by a band of white matter corpus callosum. They are also separated by a fold of dura mater falx cerebri. Each hemisphere has five lobes .

   (i) *Frontal lobe:* Possesses speech center.

   (ii) *Temporal lobe:* Possesses auditory cortex.

   (iii) *Parietal lobe:* Regulates stereognostic sensation.

   (iv) *Occipital lobe:* Regulates visual cortex.

   (v) *Limbic area:* Emotional balance.

   The surface of hemisphere has deep sulci called fissures. There are four types of fissures, i.e. central sulcus, parito–occipital sulcus, callosomargal fissure and Sylvian fissure. The covering surface is made up of grey matter known as cerebral cortex while inner part is made up of white matter containing nerve fibres.

   Functions

   (i) It controls mental activities like memory, planning, judgment and intelligence.

   (ii) Motor function

   (iii) Sensory function

   (b) **Thalamus:** There are oval mass of grey matter, situated on either side of third ventricle.

   Function: sensory relay station for the impulses.

   (c) **Basal ganglia:** It is also made up of grey matter. It consists of corpus striatum (caudate nucleus and lentiform), amygdaloid body and claustrum.

   Function: Control voluntary muscle activity.

   (d) **Hypothalamus**–It is situated below the thalamus

   Function

   (i) Synthesis of releasing factors

   (ii) Regulation of hunger, thirst, body temperature, awakefulness, obesity and gastric acid secretion.

   (iii) Synthesis of oxytocin and vasopressin.

(*Contd.*)

2. **Mid-brain**

(a) **Crus-cerebri (cerebral peduncles):** These are two fibre tracts on ventral side.

(b) **Tectum:** There are four rounded elevations called superior and inferior colliculi. They are concerned with righting reflexes.

(c) **Tegmentum:** It contains the nuclei of III, IV and V cranial nerves.

(d) **Substantial nigra:** It is made up of grey matter and is connected with corpus striatum through nigro-striatal tract. It controls muscle tone and rigidity.

(e) **Red nucleus:** It is ovoid mass of grey matter.

3. **Hind-brain (Rhombencephalon)**

(a) **Cerebellum:** It is ovoid mass having two hemispheres which are separated by a dura mater fold called falx cerebelli. A layer of dura mater called tentorium cerebelli separates it from cerebrum.

Functions

(i) Control and coordinate the skeletal muscle movement.
(ii) Maintenance of posture.

(b) **Pons:** It is situated in front of the cerebellum between the mid-brain and medulla. It contains the nuclei of Vth, VIth, VIIth and VIIIth cranial nerves.
Function: Serves as relay station.

(c) **Medulla oblongata:** It is the lower most part of the brain, showing two elevations on the ventral surface called pyramids. The nerve fibres descending from cerebrum, cross here to other side before entering the spinal cord. The crossing of nerve fibres is called decussation of pyramids. A pair of foramen of Luschka and a foramen of Magendie are found. It also contains IVth ventricles, posterior choroid plexus and nuclei of cranial nerves.

Functions

(i) *Cardiac centre:* Regulates cardiac activity
(ii) *Respiratory centre:* Controls respiration
(iii) *Vaso motor centre:* Regulation of blood pressure
(iv) *Reflex centres:* Vomiting, coughing, swallowing, sneezing, etc.

SPINAL CORD (myelon)

It is located in the vertebral canal of the vertebral column. The terminal nerve is called filum terminale and lower end of spinal cord looks like a horse tail called cauda equina.

Here the grey matter is internal, surrounds the central canal and is divided into anterior horn, posterior horn and lateral horn. The white matter is external containing nerve fibre. The 31 pairs of spinal nerves arise from it.

1. Cervical nerves - 08
2. Thoracic nerves - 12
3. Lumber nerves - 05
4. Sacral nerves - 05
5. Coccygeal nerve - 01

Functions: (i) It concerns with reflex action.
(ii) It connects the brain with other parts of the body.

...

Experiment 9

OBJECT

To study the anatomy and physiology of human **eye** with the help of chart and model.

A pair of eyes (organ of vision) is situated in orbits of the skull.

Structure: The wall of eye is made up of three coats.

1.	**Fibrous coat**	It is thick and protective coat. It has two regions: (a) **Sclera:** It is opaque and bluish white in colour. In front it forms a transparent membrane known as cornea. (b) **Cornea:** It is transparent, circular anterior one-sixth of the fibrous coat. It lacks blood vessels hence its transplantation is successful. It is slightly bulged forward.
2.	**Vascular coat**	It has three regions (a) **Choroid:** It is vascular pigmented coat and is made up of a soft connective tissue. (b) **Iris:** It is also a pigment membrane which determines the colour of the eye. There is centre aperture called pupil which contains two sets of smooth muscles, i.e. sphincters and dilators. The sphincters (circular muscle) constricts the pupil (miosis) while the dilator (radial muscle) dilates the pupil (mydriasis). (c) **Ciliary body:** The iris continues to form ciliary body which contains ciliary muscles. The suspensory ligament of lens is joined to ciliary muscle.
3.	**Inner coat (Retina)**	It is made up of four layers (a) **Pigmented layer** — it reduces the scattering of light in the eye. (b) **Receptor layer** — it contains rods and cones. (c) Bipolar nerve cells (d) Ganglion cells layer
	Macula lutea (Yellow spot)	A small area on the retina which is situated just opposite to the centre of cornea. Its middle depression is called fovea centralis. Blind spot is point in retina from where the optic nerves leave the eye ball.
	Rods and Cones	These are photo receptor cells. Rods are more than that of cones. Rods regulates twilight and night vision while cones are responsible for critical and colour vision.
	Aquous humour	Anterior chamber (in from of iris) and posterior (between iris and lens) chamber is filled with aquous humour which is secreted by ciliary processes of the ciliary body.
	Vitreous humour	A fluid filled between lens and retina.
	Lens	It is biconvex solid body which is attached by the suspensory ligament.

Working of eye

The lens along with cornea, aqueous and vitreous humour acts as focusing part. It refracts light rays passing through the eye. The image is focused on the retina. The impulse is created by rods and cones and finally it is carried through optic nerve to occipital lobe of the brain where the real perception of upright vision is experienced.

Experiment 10

OBJECT

To study the anatomy and physiology of human **ear** with the help of chart and model.

It has three parts:

1. External ear

It consists of the following organs:

(a) *Pinna:* It is an oval funnel shaped organ. It is made up of elastic cartilage. It collects sound wave.

(b) *External auditory canal:* A tube like structure contains hairs and wax glands. It continues to tympanic membrane.

(c) *Tympanic membrane (eardrum):* A thin oval membranous structure is made up of connective tissue.

2. Middle ear

It consists of tympanic cavity. It is connected with nasopharynx by a passage called the eustachian tube. It controls the air pressure of the cavity and thus protects tympanic membrane. The inner wall of tympanic cavity contains two apertures, i.e. the upper is called fenestra ovalis (oval window) and the lower is called fenestra rotendum (round window). There are three types of ear ossicles are present.

(a) *Malleus:* It is outer hammer shaped. It is attached to tympanic membrane.

(b) *Incus:* One end is connected to malleus and other is to stapes.

(c) *Stapes:* It fits into the oval window.

3. Internal ear

It has following organs

(a) *Membranous labyrinth and bony labyrinth:* Membranous labyrinth is surrounded by bony labyrinth. Both are separated by perilymphatic space which is filled with perilymph. Membrane labyrinth is also filled with a fluid called endolymph. Labyrinth consists of three structures.

(i) *Vestibule:* A sac like structure containing utricle and saccule. The vestibule bears macula of utricle and macula of saccule. A macula consists of hairs cells and supporting cells.

(ii) *Semicircular canal:* There are three semi circular canal, i.e. superior, posterior and lateral arranged at right angles to each other. Each canal has enlarged structure called ampulla. Each ampulla consists of sensory structure crista ampullaris which helps in maintenance of the equilibrium.

(iii) *Cochlea:* A long delicate coiled tube encloses into cochlear canal. The cochlear duct with cochlear canal are collectively referred as cochlea. The cochlea has three chambers -

(a) *Scala media:* Middle chamber

(b) *Scala vestibule:* Upper chamber

(c) *Scala tympani:* Lower chamber

(*Contd.*)

The middle chamber is filled with endo lymph. The floor of the scala media is called basilar membrane which bears organ of Corti. Scala vestibule and scala tympani are filled with perilymph. They are joined to each other by helicotrema.

(iv) *Organ of Corti:* It consists of receptor cells (hairs cells) and supporting cells. The supporting cells have long pillar cells and short Deiter's cells.

Physiology of hearing

The pinna receives the sound wave which is passed through external auditory canal and strike the tympanic membrane. The vibrations are transmitted to fenestra ovalis through ear ossicles. From here they are finally transmitted to organ of Corti through perilymph and endolymph. The nerve impulses are generated which is carried by VIIIth cranial nerve to the area of cerebral cortex (temporal lobe).

Equilibrium (Maintenance of balance)

1. **Dynamic equilibrium:** Cristae controls the dynamic movement. The movement of head causes bending of hairs of cristae and flow of endolymph to generate impulse which is carried to brain through VIIIth cranial nerve.
2. **Static equilibrium:** It is controlled by maculae. The change of the head or body with respect to gravity causes deflection of hair cells of maculae. They initiate nerve impulse.

3 THE TISSUES: Histology

Experiment 11

OBJECT

To study the histology of different types of tissue.

TISSUE

Tissue is the group of cells having common origin, structure and function.

Classification

It is classified as follows:

A. Epithelial tissue

B. Connective tissue

C. Muscular tissue

D. Nervous tissue

A. **Epithelial tissue:** Is made up of one or more layers of cells that provides covering or lining of the body, viscera and cavities. It is classified as.

1. Simple epithelium
2. Stratified epithelium
3. Glandular epithelium

1. **Simple epithelium:** It is made single layer of cells. It is further divided into the following:

(a) **Squamous**

(i) It is made up of single layer.

(ii) *Nature of cells:* Flat, polygonal in surface view, centrally located nucleus.

(iii) *Location:* Lungs, Bowman's capsule, inner wall of blood vessels

(iv) *Functions:* Excretion, protection, secretion and absorption.

(b) **Cuboidal epithelium**

(i) It is made up of single layer.

(ii) *Nature of cells:* Cube-like cells, polygonal .in surface view and centrally located round nucleus.

(iii) *Location:* Thyroid gland, salivary gland, bronchioles and tubules.

(iv) *Functions:* Protection, secretion and absorption.

(c) **Columnar epithelium**

(i) It is made up of single layer.

(ii) *Nature of cells:* Elongated cells, polygonal in surface view and elongated nucleus.

(*Contd.*)

Classification (Contd.)

(iii) *Location:* Stomach, intestine and gall bladder.

(iv) *Functions:* secretion and absorption.

(d) Ciliated epithelium

(i) It is made up of single layer.

(ii) *Nature of cells:* The cells may be cuboid or columnar. Cells bear hair like structures the cilia on the free surface.

(iii) Location

(a) *Cuboidal ciliated epithelium:* Urinary tubules

(b) *Columnar ciliated epithelium:* Fallopian tubes, bronchioles, etc.

2. Stratified epithelium: It is made up of several layers of cells.

(a) Stratified squamous keratinized

(i) It is made up of several layers squamous cells.

(ii) In outer few layers cytoplasm is replaced by the keratin protein.

(iii) *Nature of cells:* The superficial cells are flat and horny while lowers cells are polyhedral.

(iv) *Functions:* The horny layer prevents the loss of water and mechanical injury.

(v) *Locations:* Skin, nails and palms

(b) Stratified squamous non-keratinized

(i) It is made up of several layers of cells.

(ii) No keratinization or cornification .

(iii) *Nature of cells:* Living squamous cells.

(iv) *Functions:* Provides moderate protection.

(v) *Locations:* Buccal cavity, pharynx, vagina and oesophagus.

(c) Stratified columnar epithelium

(i) It is made up of several layers of cells.

(ii) *Nature of cells:* Elongated cells.

(iii) *Location:* Epiglottis, urethra, mammary gland and pharynx.

(d) Transitional epithelium

(i) It is made up of several layers of cells.

(ii) *Nature of cells:* Upper layer–flat cells; Lower layer pyriform and polyhedral cells

(iii) *Location:* Pelvis, ureter, urethra, bladder, etc.

(iv) *Functions:* Protection of underlying structures.

3. Glandular epithelium

(i) The glands develop from epithelial tissue.

(ii) *Function:* Secretion.

(iii) *Types*

(a) *Exocrine gland:* It may be unicellular or multicellular

a.1 *Unicellular:* e.g. goblet cells.

(*Contd.*)

Classification (Contd.)

a.2 *Multicellular:* It may be of two types.

a.2.1 *Tubular glands:* e.g. ileum.

a.2.2 *Saccular glands:* It may be simple or compound saccular glands. The simple gland is found in skin as sebaceous or oil glands. The compound gland is found in salivary gland.

(b) *Endocrine gland:* It is ductless gland. It pours its secretion in to blood.

B. Connective tissue: It is divided into three major groups:

1. Connective tissue proper: It is further divided as follow:

(a) Areolar tissue

(i) Transparent jelly like matrix is found.

(ii) It contains various types of cells like fibroblast, histiocytes, basophils, mast cells, monocytes, etc.

(iii) **Two type of fibres are present-**

a. *White fibre:* They are fine, wavy, flexible and unbranched. It is made up of collagen protein.

b. *Yellow fibre:* They are thick, straight, flexible, elastic and branched. It is made up of elastin protein.

(iv) *Function:* It connects the skin with muscle, blood vessels and nerves with the surrounding tissue. It also serves as packing materials.

(b) Adipose tissue

(i) It is made up of spherical or oval fat cells containing fat droplets and fat globules.

(ii) The fat globules occupy the most of the space of the cell pushing the nucleus and other organelles to the periphery of the cell.

(iii) *Location:* Subcutaneous, mesentery, omentum, etc.

(iv) The matrix contains fibroblasts, macrophages and fibres.

(v) *Functions*

a. Store energy and provide a definite shape to limb.

b. It protects the organs and regulates body temperature.

(c) White fibrous tissue

(i) It consists of white collagen fibres

(ii) The tissue is tough and inelastic.

(iii) It has also two forms

a. *Cords:* They are arranged a bundles, e.g. tendens which connect bones with muscles.

b. *Sheets:* The fibres form sheet like structure, e.g. pericardium, dura mater, cornea and capsule of kidney.

(d) Yellow elastic tissue

(i) It is a type of proper connective tissue.

(ii) Fibres are thicker, branched and yellow in colour.

(Contd.)

Classification (Contd.)

(iii) They are straight, flexible, elastic and occur singly.
(iv) They are made up of elastin protein.
(v) They are found in two forms, i.e. cords and sheet.
(vi) *Location:* Lungs, wall of blood vessels, bronchioles, etc.
(vii) *Functions:* It helps in movement of organs and in expiration.

(e) Reticular tissue

(i) It consists of reticular cells and reticular fibres.
(ii) The reticular fibres are thinner than white fibres and branched.
(iii) It is a member of reticuloendothelial system.
(iv) It is made up of reticulin protein.
(v) *Location:* Spleen, lymph gland, liver, bone marrow, etc.
(vi) *Functions:* The cells are phagocytic and provide defence to the body.

2. Skeletal tissue

(a) Cartilage
(b) Bone

3. Vascular tissue

(a) Blood
(b) Lymph

C. Muscular tissue: The muscle tissue originates from embryonic mesoderm. The muscle cell is called myocytes. They are of three types.

1. Striated muscle

(i) It is also called skeletal muscle. Because it is attached to the bone.
(ii) Shape — cylindrical.
(iii) Multinucleate.
(iv) Striations (alternate light and dark band) are present.
(v) Sarcoplasmic reticulum is well developed.
(vi) Intercalated disc — Absent.
(vii) It gets fatigue soon.
(viii) Voluntary in function.
(ix) They are innervated by motor nerves.
(x) Blood supply is abundant.
(xi) *Location:* Body wall and limb.

2. Non-striated muscle

(i) It is also called smooth, visceral and involuntary muscle.
(ii) Shape — spindle.
(iii) Uninucleate, nucleus at the centre.
(iv) Striations (alternate light and dark band) are absent.
(v) Sarcoplasmic reticulum is less developed.

(Contd.)

Classification (Contd.)

(vi) No intercalated disc.

(vii) They are not fatigued soon. They contract slowly for a long time.

(viii) Involuntary in function.

(ix) They are innervated by ANS.

(x) Location: Visceral organs like GIT, blood vessel, urinary bladder, ciliary body, etc.

3. **Cardiac muscle**

(i) This tissue forms three dimensional network.

(ii) Shape — short and cylindrical.

(iii) Uninucleate, nucleus at the centre.

(iv) Myofibrils distinct with faint light and dark band.

(v) Sarcoplasmic reticulum is less developed.

(vi) Intercalated disc is present.

(vii) Rhythmic contraction.

(viii) Involuntary in function.

(ix) They are innervated by ANS and CNS both.

(x) *Location:* Heart.

(xi) Blood supply is abundant.

4. **Nervous tissue**

(i) Nerves cells are called neuron

(ii) It is a structural and functional unit of the nervous system.

(iii) Cell body (Cyton) consists of neuroplasm, nucleus, mitochondria and Golgi bodies.

(iv) The cell process are of two types:

(a) *Dendrons (dendrites):* These are much branched processes for receiving impulses.

(b) *Axon:* A single long cylindrical process for conducting impulses away from the cyton.

(v) The nerve fibres are of two types, i.e. myelinated and non myelinated.

(vi) The myelinated nerve fibre has node of Ranvier which help in rapid transmission of nerve impulses.

(vii) The neurilemma consists of Schwann's cells which produce the myelin sheath around the neuraxis.

(viii) *Neuroglia:* It is supporting and packing cells found in brain, spinal cord and ganglia.

(ix) Function

(a) To serve and transmit the impulses.

(b) Coordination and integration of the various activities of the body.

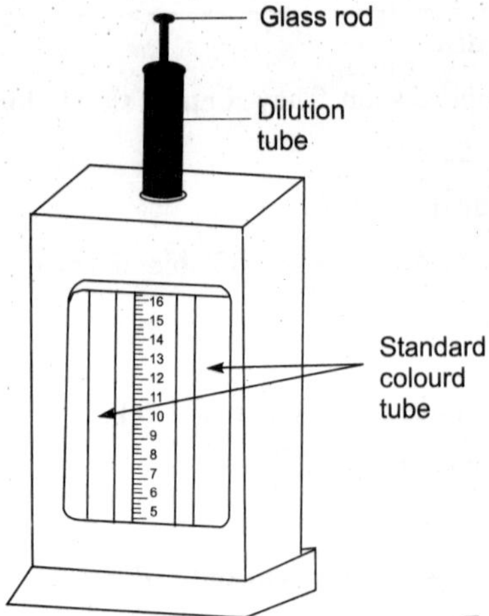

Haemoglobinometer

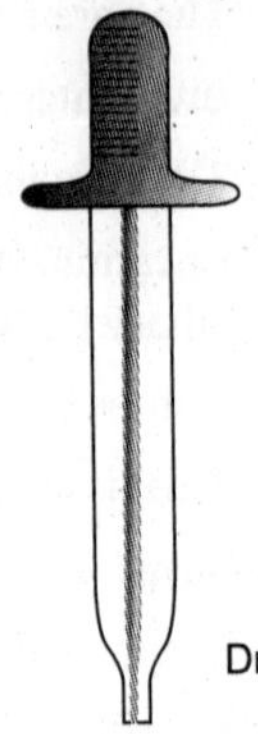

Dropper

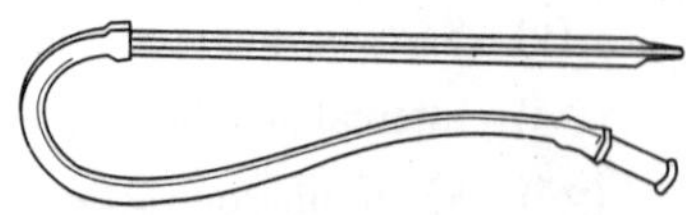

20 cu mm micropipette

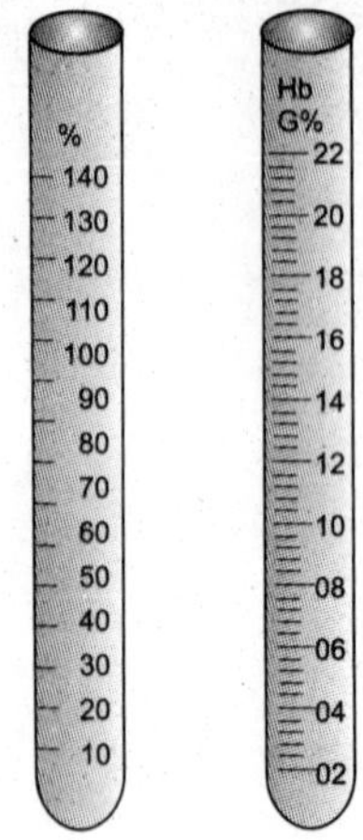

A B

Dilutrion tube

4 HAEMATOLOGY

Experiment 12

OBJECT

Estimation of haemoglobin (Hb).

Chemicals

N/10 HCl, distilled water and sprit.

Principle

Haemoglobin is a colouring, respiratory pigment, made up of haem and globin protein. The estimation of haemoglobin involves its reaction with 0.1 N HCl to form acid haematin which colour is compared against a pair of standard colour glass. The above method of determination of haemoglobin is called (visual method) Shali's method. The other methods are photoelectric, chemical; specific gravity method, etc. one gram of haemoglobin is equivalent to 1.34 cc of oxygen. Haemoglobin content is reported in gram percentage. Thus oxygen carrying capacity also can be reported. The haemoglobin determination has diagnostic value. The haemoglobin content higher than normal is seen in polycythemia while in anaemia its content is lower than the normal value. The haemoglobin helps in transport of oxygen and carbon dioxide, maintenance of pH and ions and formation of bile.

Normal value of haemoglobin

Sex	Grams per 100 ml of blood
Men	14–18
Women	12–16
Infants	14 - 20

Procedure

Keep the apparatus dry and clean. Fill the graduated dilution tube (up to mark 2 on gram % marking) with N/10 HCl. The left ring finger is cleaned with rectified sprit. Then prick the left ring finger with the sterilized needle. The blood is sucked in the haemometer pipette exactly up to 20 cm mark. The blood is transferred to dilution tube containing N/10 HCl. The distilled water is added drop wise drop until the colour of the solution matches with the standard colour glass. The value of haemoglobin content is noted is gram per 100 ml of blood as well as in percentage too.

Result

Patient name
Age
Sex
Haemoglobin content ------ gram %
Haemoglobin content ------- %
Date

Experiment 13

OBJECT

To report clotting time of your blood.

Principle

Clotting time

It is the time interval in between onset of bleeding to form a clot. The blood clot formation stops bleeding. The platelets play an important role to initiate clotting of the blood. There are 13 clotting factors that take part in process of clotting. It takes place in the following steps-

1. Activation of prothrombin
2. Conversion of prothrombin in to thrombin.
3. Conversion of fibrinogen to fibrin (clot).

Normal range 3–4 minutes

Procedure

The left ring finger is cleaned with rectified sprit. Then prick the left ring finger with the sterilized needle. The capillary glass tube is taken and the blood is sucked in to a capillary tube. The small piece of capillary tube is broken at every 15 seconds until a fine thread of clot is seen. The time interval in between the appearance of the drop of the blood and the thread of blood clot is taken as clotting time.

Result

Patient's name

Age

Sex

Clotting time

Date

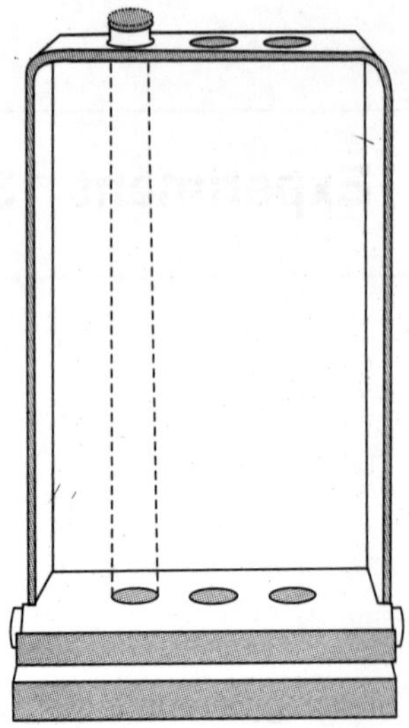

Sedimentation rate rack

Experiment 14

OBJECT

To report ESR of your blood.

PRINCIPLE

Erythrocyte sedimentation rate (ESR)

The rate at which erythrocytes settle down or millimetre (mm) of clear plasma formed at the top of vertical column in an hour is called ESR. The blood is mixed with anticoagulant. It is allowed to stand in a vertical tube. There are two methods which is widely used for determining the ESR.

1. *Westergren's method:* This tube is graduated in mm up to 200 mm mark and is opened at both ends.
2. *Wintrobe's method:* This tube is graduated in mm up to 100 mark and is opened at the top and closed at the bottom.

The ESR has diagnostic value in many diseases and physiological conditions.

Increased sedimentation rate: Tuberculosis, cancer, rheumatic fever anaemia, menstruation, pregnancy and leukaemia.

Decreased ESR: Congestive heart failure, polycythaemia, congenital diseases.

Normal range (ESR)

Method	Men mm per hour	Women mm per hour
Westergren	0–15 mm	0–20 mm
Wintrobe	0–9 mm	0–20 mm

Procedure

Take anticoagulant solution (1/5th of the blood), i.e. oxalate or citrate in a clean dry vial and withdraw two cc of blood by vein-puncture. Mix the blood with anticoagulant solution properly. Then blood is sucked into Westergren tube up to 200 mark and it was placed in the stand. The Westergren tube must be held vertically in the stand. The reading is noted after one hour.

Result

Patient's name
Age
Sex
ESR value
Date

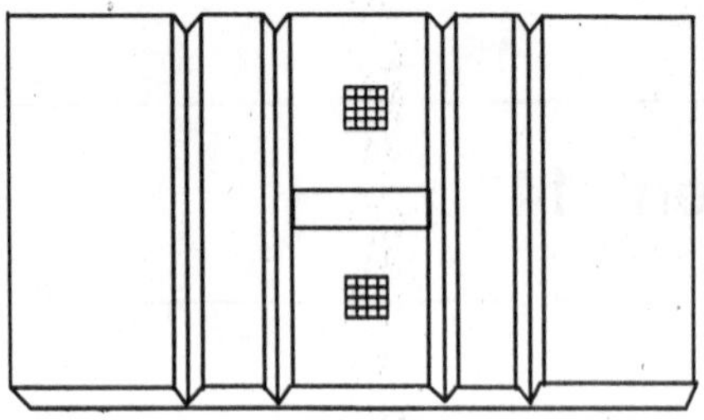

Neubaur's counting slip

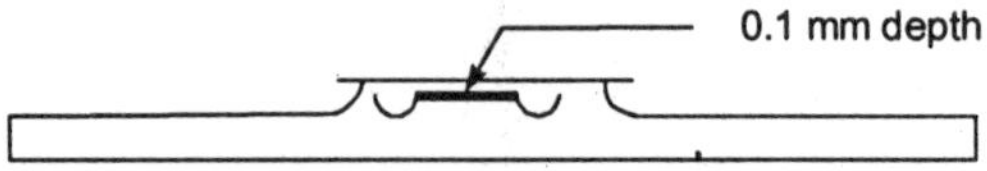

Neubaur's counting chamber showing depth on keeping coverslip

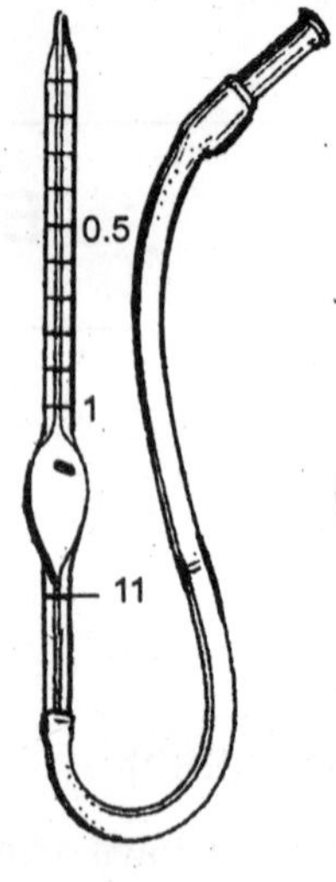

W.B.C.Pipette

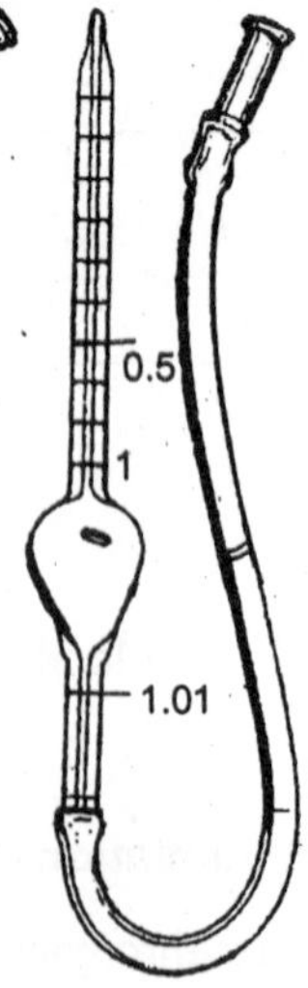

RBC micropipette

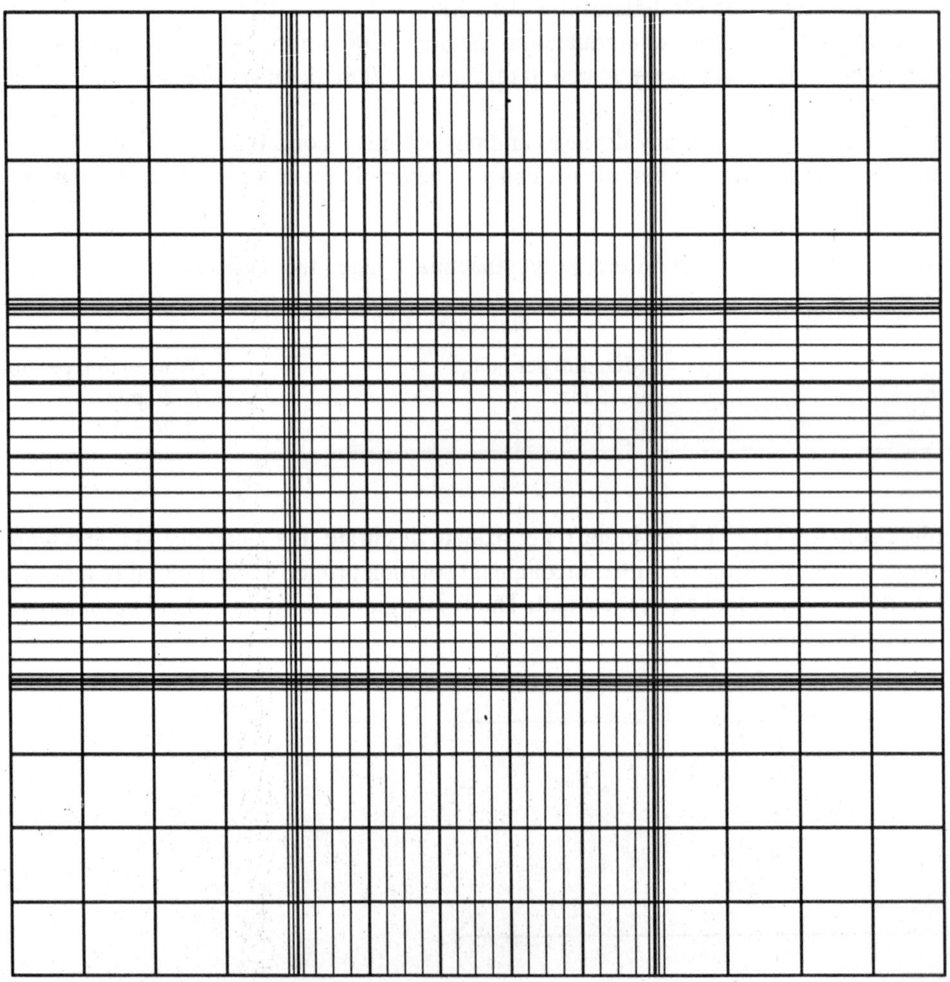

Neubaur's counting chamber (magnified)

***Fig. Exp.* 15.1**

Experiment 15

OBJECT

To report TLC of your blood.

Apparatus

Microscope, sterilized needle, haemocytometer, cotton, etc.

Chemicals

Sprit and WBC diluting fluid.

WBC Diluting Fluid

Gentian violet (1%)	–	1 ml
Glacial acetic	–	2 ml
Distilled water	–	qs 100 ml

Principle

The leucocytes count is the number of WBC. Present in one cubic millimetre of blood. The leucocytes are of two types.

1. *Granular:* Neutrophil, acidophil, basophil.
2. *Agranular:* Lymphocytes, monocytes.

The WBC play an important role in body defence mechanism against invading microbes by phagocytosis. They also help in antibody formation. Normal WBC range, 4000–11000 per cubic mm of blood.

Leucocytosis: Increased number of WBC than normal, e.g. pneumonia, tonsillitis, diphtheria, rheumatic fever, etc.

Leucopenia: Decreased number of WBC than normal, e.g. influenza, typhoid, hepatitis, cirrhosis of liver, myxoedema, etc.

Haemocytometer: It consists of RBC pipette, WBC Pipette, Neuber counting chamber and cover slip.

WBC pipette: There are three graduation marks on the pipette, i.e. 0.5, 1 (just below the bulb) and 11 (just at the top of the bulb). There is a bulb containing white bead which helps in mixing and diluting the blood.

Neuber counting chamber: There are two ruled areas separated by groove. The four corner squares (1 mm × 1 mm × 0.1 mm) are used for WBC count as shown in Fig. Exp. 15.1 (on facing page).

Procedure

The finger-tip is treated with rectified sprit and let it be dry. The left finger-tip is pricked with sterilized needle and the blood is sucked exactly up to 0.5 mark. The diluting fluid is taken in watch glass and this blood is sucked up to 11 mark. The pipette is shaken for proper mixing. Then for charging of chamber with diluted blood, discard the first 3 to 4 drops of diluted blood and place the cover slip on ruled area of the slide. The diluted blood (1 drop) is placed at the edge of cover slip. The diluted fluid is spread uniformly by capillary action. Trapping of air bubbles are avoided. It is left for 5 minutes for the cells to settle town. Focus the microscope at low power (10 × 10) and count the WBC in the four big WBC squares. The adjustment of light by the diaphragm and mirror is essential for clear vision of cells to be examined.

Calculation	Volume of 1 big square	=	1 × 1 × 0.1
		=	0.1 cu mm
	Volume of 4 big square	=	4 × 0.1 cu mm
		=	0.4 cu mm
	Since 0.4 cu mm blood	=	N number of WBC cells
	So 1 cu mm blood	=	N/0.4 of WBC cells
	Here dilution factor	=	20
	So 1 cu mm of undiluted blood	=	N/0.4 × 20 of WBC cells
		=	N × 50
	Where N is the total number of WBC cells in four big squares.		

Result

Patient's name

Age

Sex

TLC

Date

Experiment 16

OBJECT

To report DLC (differential leucocytes count).

Principle

The leucocytes is of two types.

1. *Granulocytes:* Granules are found in cytoplasm, e.g. neutrophil, eosinophil, basophil.
2. *Agranulocytes:* Granules are absent, e.g. lymphocytes and monocytes.

When the blood smear after drying is fixed and stained by acid and basic dye, leucocytes are differentiated to identify the each variety so that each one can be counted.

Neutrophil

Stain	-	By neutral dye
% count	-	55–70%
Size	-	10–12 μ
Nucleus	-	2–5 lobed
Cytoplasm	-	Fine pink or violet granules

Eosinophil

Stain	-	By acid dye
% count	-	2–4%
Size	-	10–12 μ
Nucleus	-	Two lobed
Cytoplasm	-	Coarse red colour granules

Basophil

Stain	-	By basic dye
% count	-	0.5%
Size	-	8–10 μ
Nucleus	-	Indistinct
Cytoplasm	-	coarse blue colour granules

Lymphocyte

Stain	-	Nucleus takes blue stain
% count	-	20–35%
Size	-	Small 8–10 μ, Large 10–15 μ
Nucleus	-	Round
Cytoplasm	-	No granules

Monocyte

Stain	-	Faint blue stain or grey
% count	-	2–4%
Size	-	18 μ
Nucleus	-	Eccentric, notched
Cytoplasm	-	No granules

Apparatus and Reagent

Leishman's stain, glass slide, distilled water, microscope, cotton, rectified spirit and needle.

Procedure

The finger is cleaned and pricked to get a free flow of blood. A drop of blood is taken on the side of a slide. A blood smear is prepared by the help of other slide. The Leishman's stain (8–10 drops) is added to the dried film. It is allowed to stand for one minute. Then it is diluted with an equal amount of distilled water. It is left for 8–10 minutes. It is washed with running water. The film is dried in air. The film is examined under forty power and oil immersion objective lens. The counting should be done for whole of the film and percentage count of each type of the cell is recorded.

Observation

S. No.	*Types of cell*	*Count*	*Total count*	*% count*
1.	Neutrophils			
2.	Eosinophils			
3.	Basophils			
4.	Monocytes			
5.	Lymphocytes			

Result

Name of the patient	-	
Age	-	
Sex	-	
Neutrophils	-	%
Eosinophils	-	%
Basophils	-	%
Monocytes	-	%
Lymphocytes	-	%

Various stages of malarial parasite

	P. falciparum malignant tertian	*P. vivax benign tertian*	*P. malariae benign quartan*	*P. ovale benign tertian*
Schizogony Cycle hours	48 hours/under	48 hours	72 hours	48 hours
Trophozoite	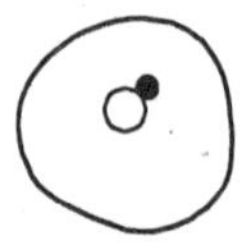	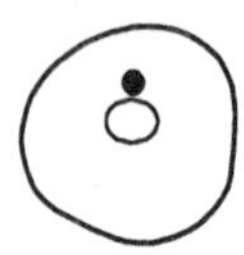	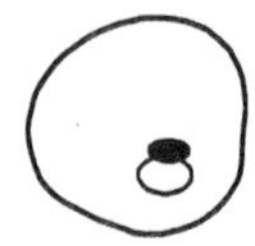	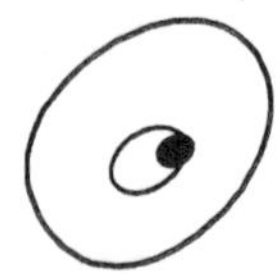
(a) Early	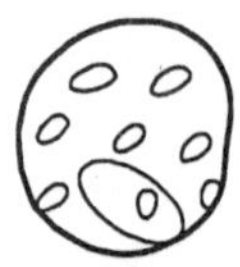	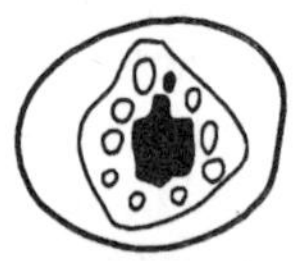	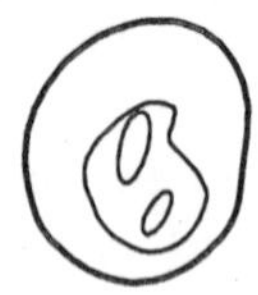	
(b) Intermediate	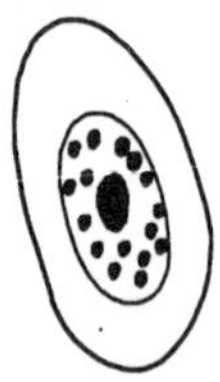	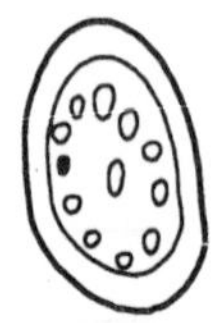	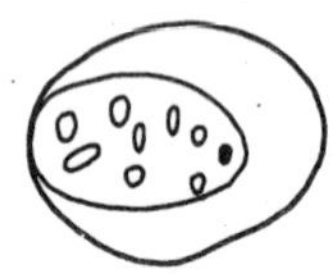	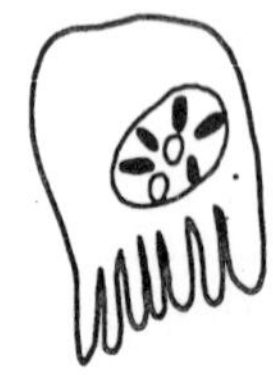
(c) Late				
Matured Schizont	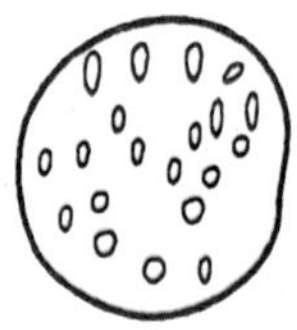	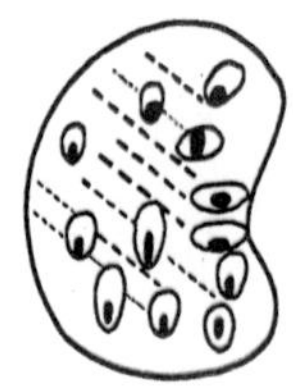	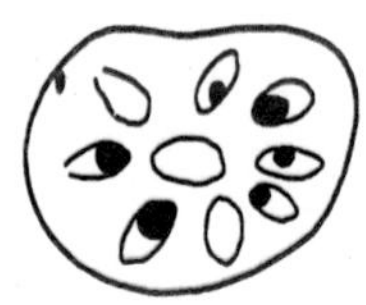	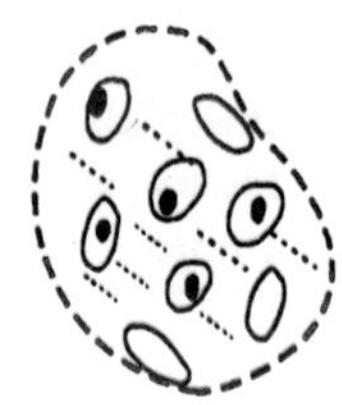
No. of merozoites	18–24	12–24	6–12	6–12
Gametocyte	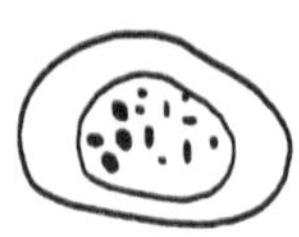	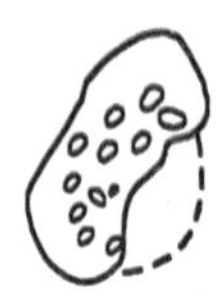	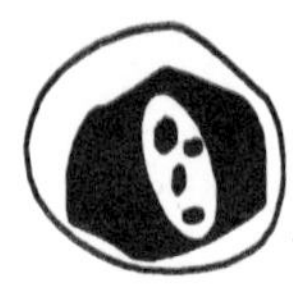	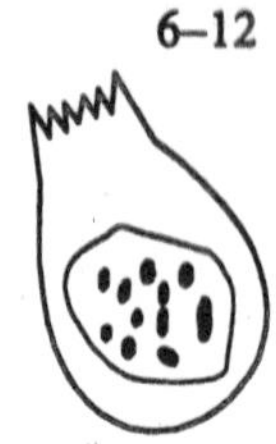
	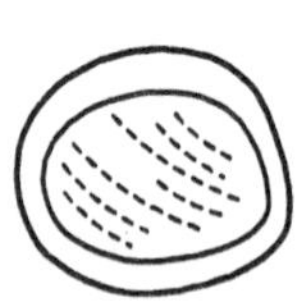	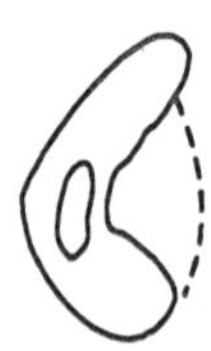	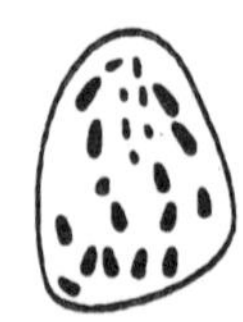	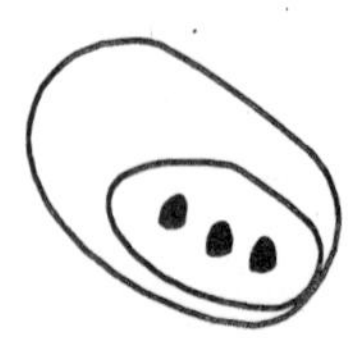

Experiment 17

OBJECT

Examination of blood smear for **malaria parasite.**

Principle

Malaria fever is caused by protozoon parasite:

Plasmodium falciparum (*Pf*)
Plasmodium malariae (*Pm*)
Plasmodium vivax (*Pv*)
Plasmodium ovale (*Po*)

This parasite has two hosts, i.e. female anopheles mosquito and man.

Morphology of Malaria Parasites

TROPHOZOITES

Character	*PV*	*Pm*	*Pf*	*Po*
Shape	delicate ring	compact ring	delicate ring	dense ring
Pigment	absent	may be present	absent	absent
Chromatin	fine dot sometimes two in number	inform of mass, in side ring	fine dots two in number	dense with well-defined mass

DEVELOPING TROPHOZOITES

Pigment colour	Yellow brown	Dark brown	Black	Dark yellow brown
Quantity of pigment	Medium	Abundant	Medium	Medium

SCHIZONTS

Mature merozoites range	14–24	6–12	8–32	6–12
Size	Medium	Large	Small	Large
Pigment	Yellow brown	Dark brown	Black	Dark yellow brown

GAMETOCYTES

Size of microgametocytes	Round or oval	Round compact	Kidney shaped (crescent)	Round compact
Number of macrogameto-cytes in blood smear	Many	Scanty	Many	Scanty

Procedure

Blood film is prepared. Preparation and staining technique is similar to that of DLC. After staining the blood smear, one drop of immersion oil is put on it and is examined under oil immersion objective. The different species of malaria parasite is identified by their morphological character of trophozoites, schizonts and gametocytes.

Result

MP–Positive/Negative

If positive, type of species should be reported.

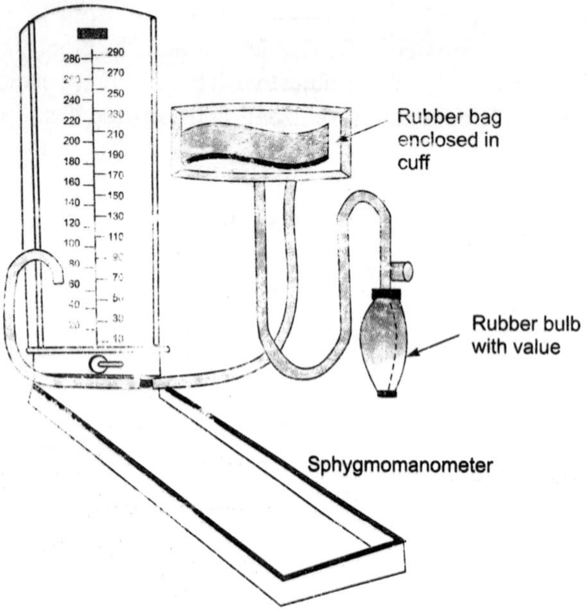

Sphygmomanometer

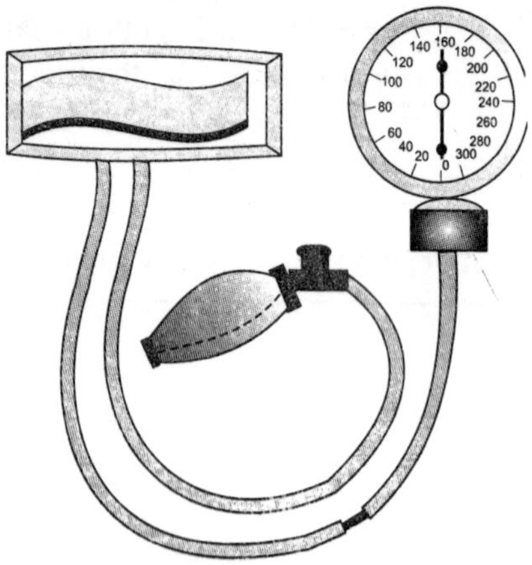

Sphygmomanometer-aneroid type

5 OTHER PROCEDURES

Experiment 18

OBJECT

Recording of **blood pressure** (ausculatory method).

Apparatus

Sphygmomanometer, stethoscope.

Principle

The blood pressure of the bronchial artery is balanced against the air pressure of rubber cuff around the brachial artery. The pressure is recorded by instrument known as sphygmomanometer.

Blood pressure

It is the lateral pressure exerted by blood on the wall of blood vessels.

Systolic pressure

It is the maximum pressure that is exerted during the systole of the heart.

Diastolic pressure

It is the minimum pressure that is exerted during the diastole of the heart.

Pulse pressure

The difference between the two (systolic and diastolic pressure) in known as pulse pressure.

Blood pressure	-	Normal range (adult)
Systolic	-	100–145 mm of Hg
Diastolic	-	60–90 mm of Hg.
Average	-	120/80 mm Hg

Physiological variations are being shown for systolic blood pressure only by the following factors, e.g. age, climate, sex, body build, posture, sleep, stress and hormones. Variations in diastolic pressure has great clinical significance. Increase in diastolic pressure is the indicative that the heart is going towards failure.

Procedure

The individual is allowed to sit on a chair in relax condition. The cuff of the instrument is tied round the arm. The pressure in the cuff is raised above the systolic pressure (200 mm). The chest piece of the stethoscope is placed over the brachial artery. Then the pressure is lowered gradually. As a result blood begins to flow through compressed artery in the distal segment. It creates a clear, sharp, tapping sound. The label of the mercury in the manometer is recorded. This indicates the systolic pressure. The air pressure continues to fall and loud sound fades rapidly. This indicates diastolic pressure.

Result

Systolic blood pressure	-	--------- mm Hg.
Diastolic blood pressure	-	--------- mm Hg.

Experiment 19

OBJECT

Recording of pulse rate, heart rate and body temperature.

Apparatus

Clinical thermometer, stethoscope .

Principle

Pulse rate: Pulse is the pressure changes transmitted in the form of a wave of the arterial walls. Pulse rate is same as heart rate. The radial artery of the wrist is very superficial that can be felt easily. It is important clinically to examine the condition of the heart, arteries and blood pressure. A high pulse rate is reported in new born babies, female, emotion, excitement, etc.

Heart rate

Heart rate is regulated by ANS. The parasympathetic has inhibitory effect while the sympathetic system has excitatory effect. It normally varies with respiration, temperature, exercise, oxygen lack and blood pressure.

Heart rate	-	Normal range
Foetus	-	140–150 per minute
Child	-	100–110 per minute
Adult	-	70–80 per minute

Temperature

The body temperature is maintained by thermoregulatory mechanism. The hypothalamus plays an important role in regulation of body temperature. The respiration and circulation also help in this process. The elevated body temperature is called fever. Hyperpyrexia causes local bleeding and degeneration of cells leading to death.

Temperature	-	Normal range
Oral	-	97–99° F (36–37.2° C)
Rectal	-	1° F greater than oral temperature

Procedure

Pulse rate: The radial artery of the wrist is palpated by pressing it and the pulse rate is recorded for 1 minute.

Heart rate: The heart rate is noted by placing the chest piece of a stethoscope against the location of the heart for 1 minute.

Temperature

Body temperature is noted by placing the bulb of the clinical thermometer in axilla or in mouth. The rise in mercury column is the indicative of the body temperature.

Result

Pulse rate	-
Heart rate	-
Body temperature	-

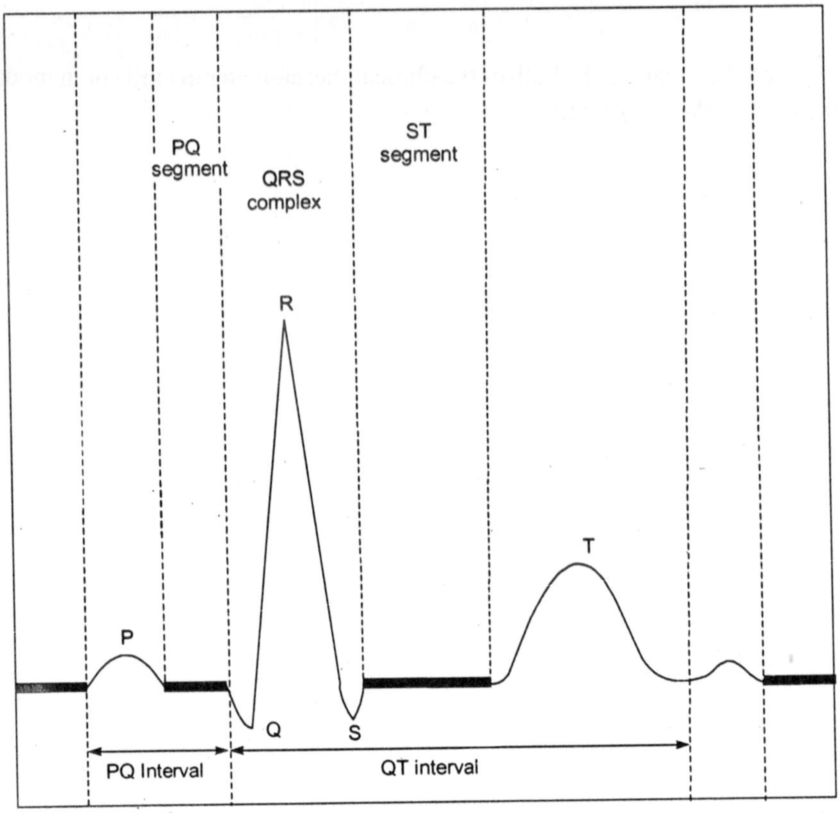
PQ
segment
QRS
complex
ST
segment
R
T
P
Q
S
PQ Interval
QT interval

Experiment 20

OBJECT

Recording of ECG.

Apparatus

ECG machine.

Principle

Graphical tracing of electrical activity during the cardiac cycle is called electrocardiogram (ECG), and the machine by which the ECG is recorded is known as electrocardiograph.

This recording is done through string galvanometer or moving coil galvanometer. The pair of connections between the two parts of the body is called lead. The following types of lead is used.

1. **Standard limb leads:** The connections are made as follow.

Lead	Negative terminal	Positive terminal
I.	Right arm	Left arm
II.	Right arm	Left leg
III.	Left arm	Left leg

2. **Augmented unipolar limb leads:** These are three types of leads known as aVR, aVL and aVF
   aVR: The right arm is connected to positive terminal while the left arm and left leg to the negative terminals.
   aVL: Similarly the left arm is connected to the positive terminals and the rest two parts to negative terminals.
   aVF: The left leg is connected to the positive terminal and the rest two parts to negative terminals.
3. **Chest leads (Unipolar):** There are six chest leads represented as V1, V2, V3, V4, V5 and V6.
   V1: IVth intercostal space slightly away from the right sternal border.
   V2: IVth intercostal space slightly away from the left sternal border.
   V3: Mid point between V2 and V4.
   V4: Vth intercostal space at left mid clavicular line.
   V5: Vth intercostal space in anterior axillary line.
   V6: Mid axillary line intersects perpendicular at the level of V4.

Interpretation

P wave is called atrial complex.

QRST is called ventricular complex.

P: It is first upward deflection. The average duration is about 0.1 sec. It indicates about the conductivity of cardiac muscles.

QRST (Ventricular complex): It shows ventricular depolarisation. The average duration of QRST is 0.43 sec. and QRS should be less than 0.08 sec.

Q: It is negative wave and is produced by the activity of the septum.

R: It is the first tallest positive deflection of ventricular origin.

S: It is downward deflection.

T: It is the last upward deflection of an average duration of 0.27 sec. It shows the ventricular repolarisation.

U: It is often due to slow repolarisation.

The standard limb leads indicates the functional abnormalities of heart. It is useful for diagnosis of arrhythmias.

Augmented unipolar limb leads determine the position of heart and also indicates the extent of ventricular damage while chest leads is the indicative of the bundle block as well as the ventricular position.

Viva Voce

Q1. Name one organ in human body which has both exocrine and endocrine parts.
Ans. Pancreas.

Q2. Name the vitamin required for formation of rhodopsin.
Ans. Vitamin A.

Q3. Which is the largest gland in our body?
Ans. Liver.

Q4. What is micelles ?
Ans. The end product of fat, i.e. fatty acid, glycerol are incorporated into small water soluble droplets called micelles with help of bile salt and phospholipids.

Q5. Name the different parts of large intestine of human.
Ans. Caecum, colon and rectum.

Q6. What is enamel of teeth made of?
Ans. Calcium phosphate.

Q7. Define peristalsis.
Ans. A wave of constrictions produced by the involuntary contraction of smooth muscles of GIT.

Q8. How does the human adult digest milk protein?
Ans. Milk proteins are digested by rennin into stomach and by chemotrypsin in the intestine.

Q9. Define external respiration.
Ans. Uptake of oxygen from the surrounding medium and elimination of carbon dioxide.

Q10. What is internal respiration?
Ans. Uptake of oxygen, oxidation of nutrient (glucose) and released of carbon dioxide.

Q11. What is inspiration and expiration?
Ans. Inspiration–Breathing in air is called inspiration and breathing out of carbon dioxide is called expiration

Q12. Define tidal volume and vital capacity.
Ans. The tidal volume of air inspired and expired during normal process of breathing.
Vital capacity is the volume of air that is breathed out by maximum expiration after taking maximum inspiration.

Q13. What term is used for the volume of air left into lungs even after the most powerful expiration?
Ans. Residual volume.

Q14. Write the role of diaphragm in respiration.
Ans. Diaphragm increases the volume of thoracic cavity as a result of its contraction of muscles and also decreases the air pressure. Thus inspiration takes place. When diaphragm relaxes expiration takes place.

Q15. Write in proper sequence the organs concern with respiration in human.
Ans. Nostril ⟶ Nasal cavity ⟶ Nasopharynx ⟶ Larynx ⟶ trachea ⟶ Bronchi ⟶ bronchioles ⟶ Alveoli.

Q16. How does lung expend and contract?
Ans. The downward and upward movement of the diaphragm lengthens and shortens the chest cavity. Similarly the elevation and depression of the ribs, increase or decrease of the volume of the chest cavity.

Q17. Write the name of the respiratory regulatory center of the brain?
Ans. Medulla oblongata ⟶ inspiratory center and expiratory center
Pons ⟶ Pneumotaxic center and apneustic center.

Q18. Define cardiac cycle.

Ans. The sequence of events take place during a heart beat.

Q19. What is myogenic heart?

Ans. In the heart cardiac impulses are self generated and it is not brought to heart by any nerve fibre.

Q20. What is SA node? What is other name of it?

Ans. It is sino-atrial node. It is also called pace maker.

Q21. How is first heart sound produced?

Ans. The first heart sound is produced by the closure of AV valves at the start of ventricular systole.

Q22. What is electrocardiogram (ECG). Write its significance.

Ans. It is graphical representation of the electrical potential changes produced by the cardiac muscles during cardiac cycle as a function of time. Deviations from the normal pattern indicates the heart disease.

Q23. Differentiate between the artery and vein.

Ans.

S. No.	*Artery*	*Vein*
1.	Flow of blood away from heart.	Flow of blood toward the heart.
2.	Thick wall	Thin wall
3.	No valves	Valves present
4.	Located deep in tissue	Located superficially
5.	It carries oxygenated blood except pulmonary artery	It carries deoxygenated blood except pulmonary vein

Q24. What is artificial pace-maker?

Ans. It is an electronic device which is implanted subcutaneously which controls the rhythmicity of the heart, when natural pace maker (SA Node) fail to function.

Q25. Write the name of different part tubules of kidney.

Ans. (a) Proximal convoluted tubule
(b) Loop of Henle
  (i) Descending limb
  (ii) Ascending limb
(c) Distal convoluted tubules

Q26. Write the name of structural and functional unit of a kidney.

Ans. Nephron.

Q27. What is micturition?

Ans. It is the act of voiding urine.

Q28. Write the name of processes involved in the formation of urine.

Ans. (a) Glomerular filtration
(b) Tubular reabsorption
(c) Tubular secretion
(d) Tubular synthesis

Q29. What is vasa rectae?

Ans. The efferent arteriole gives rise to some parallel, wide and thin-walled straight capillaries called vasa-rectae that lie close to loop of Henle.

Q30. What is nephritis, uraemia and albuminuria?

Ans. *Nephritis:* Inflammation of glomeruli of nephrons.
Uraemia: Presence of excess urea in urine.
Albuminuria: Presence of albumin in urine.

Q.31. Define haemodialysis.

Ans. It is the process of removing the excess urea from the blood of patient suffering from renal failure, using an artificial kidney.

Q32. What is juxtaglomerular apparatus? Write its functions.

Ans. It is a multi-hormonal rennin-angiotensin aldosterone system found in afferent arteriole. It responses to decrease in blood pressure or blood volume in the afferent arteriole. It releases renin which converts angiotensionogen into angiotensin II. As a result the blood pressure is increased.

Q33. How many polar bodies are given out in production of one egg?

Ans. Two.

Q34. How many ova will be produced by mature oocyte?

Ans. One.

Q35. Where does fertilization take place in human female?

Ans. Fallopian tube.

Q36. Name the enzyme of the sperm releases at the time of fertilization.

Ans. Hyaluronidase.

Q37. What is spermatogenesis?

Ans. It is the process of formation spermatozoa.

Q38. Define zygote.

Ans. The fertilized ovum is called zygote.

Q39. What is endometrium?

Ans. The lining layer of uterus is called endometrium.

Q40. Define ovulation.

Ans. The rapture of mature Graafian follicle and release of ovum from it is called ovulation.

Q41. Define placenta.

Ans. It is the temporary association between the foetus and maternal tissues.

Q42. Where are Leydig cells located? What do they secrete?

Ans. These are located in the connective tissue of testis, inbetween the seminiferous tubules. They secrete testosterone.

Q43. What is clone? Name two animals that has been cloned.

Ans. Clone is a population of genetically identical individuals resulting from single parent, e.g. boar calf and dolly.

Q44. Explain the role of the following hormones with reference to menstrual cycle.
FSH, LH, estrogen and progesterone.

Ans. **FSH:** It stimulates the growth of follicles and the maturation of an ovum in it during proliferative phase. It also stimulates the secretion of estrogens.

LH: It stimulates ovulation. It induces the formation of corpus luteum and also stimulates secretion of progesterone.

Estrogen: It controls and regulates the secondary sex organs of female. The endometrium thickens and the contraction of uterine muscles increase.

Progesterone: It brings about the pregnancy changes. It prevents ovulation. It also controls the growth of mammary glands.

Q45. Which part of the ear functions for maintaining body balance?

Ans. Utricle, saccule and semicircular canals.

Q46. Define reflex action.

Ans. It is defined as a spontaneous, involuntary, nerve-mediated activity produced at the unconscious level.

Q47. Define accommodation.

Ans. It is a reflex mechanism by which light rays from objects at various locations in near vision are brought to focus on the retina.

Q48. What is organ of Corti?
Ans. It is the smallest unit of the ear made up of the basilar membrane, sensory hair cells and tectorial membrane.

Q49. Name the three bones in sequence forming the auditory ossicles .
Ans. Malleus, incus and stapes. These are located in middle ear.

Q50. Differentiate between rods and cones.
Ans.

S. No.	*Rods*	*Cones*
1.	More sensitive to light and are meant for vision in dim light.	These are meant for vision in bright light.
2.	Do not have ability to make colour image.	Ability to make colour image.
3.	They contain rhodopsin.	They contain iodopsin.

Q51. What is the diagnostic importance of estimation of haemoglobin?
Ans. In anaemia haemoglobin content is low than that of normal while in polycythemia its value rises.

Q52. What are different methods for estimation of haemoglobin?
Ans. (a) Chemical method
(b) Colorimetric method
(c) Specific gravity method

Q53. What is leucocyctosis and leucopenia?
Ans. WBC count is more than normal is termed as leucocytosis while its count is less than normal is called leucopenia.

Q54. Write the composition of WBC diluting fluid?
Ans. Glacial acetic acid — 3 ml
Gentian violet (1%) — 1 ml
Distilled water q.s. — 100 ml

Q55. What is neutrophilia and eosinophilia? Write their diagnostic importance.
Ans. Increase count of neutrophils is called neutrophilia and eosinophils is called eosinophilia. Increase in count of neutrophils is found in pneumonia, meningitis, tonsillitis, leukemia, etc. Similarly increase in count of eosinophils is seen in asthma, skin diseases, hay fever, etc.

Q56. Write diagnostic importance of monocytes and lymphocytes.
Ans. Monocytosis (Increase in number of monocytes) is found in tuberculosis, typhoid, leukemia, etc. while lymphocytosis (increase in number of lymphocytes) is found in whooping cough and leukemia.

Q57. Write diagnostic significance of ESR.
Ans. Increase in value of ESR is observed in the following diseases like rheumatic fever, pneumonia, cancer, syphilis, tuberculosis, leukemia, anaemia, menstruation, etc.

Q58. What is hypertension?
Ans. The word hypertension is used for increase in arterial blood pressure.

Q59. What is systolic and diastolic blood pressure?
Ans. Systolic blood pressure: It is the maximum blood pressure during the contraction of the heart.
Diastolic blood pressure: It is the minimum blood pressure during the relaxation of the heart.

Q60. What are the factors effecting blood pressure?
Ans. Cardiac output, viscosity of blood, elasticity of blood vessels, blood volume and peripheral resistance.

Q61. Enlist the different leads that are used conventionally.
Ans. (a) Standard limb leads
(b) Chest leads
(c) Augmented unipolar limb leads

Q62. What is tachycardia and bradycardia?

Ans. *Tachycardia:* Increase in heart rate than the normal value.
Bradycardia: Decrease in heart rate than the normal value.

Q63. Write the harmful effect of high temperature on the human body.

Ans. High temperature causes the degeneration of cells throughout the body and may lead to local bleeding. The brain cells are greatly influenced.

Q64. Give examples of the following bones:
Long bone, short bone, flat bone, irregular bone and sesamoid bone.

Ans.

Long bone	Femur, humerus
Short bone	Wrist, ankle
Flat bone	Scapula, pelvic
Irregular bone	Face bone and vertebrae
Sesamoid bone	Patella

Q65. Write the causative microorganism of malaria fever.

Ans. The malaria fever is caused by protozoon parasite:
Plasmodium vivax
Plasmodium malariae
Plasmodium ovale
Plasmodium falciparum

Q66. Write the name of the hosts of *Plasmodium*.

Ans. Female anopheles mosquito and human.

Q67. Which species of *Plasmodium* is regarded more fatal and dangerous in India?

Ans. *Plasmodium falciparum*